25 Organic Belly Fat Burner Recipes

Disclaimer and Terms of Use:

Effort has been made to ensure that the information in this book is accurate and complete, however, the author and the publisher do not warrant the accuracy of the information, text and graphics contained within the book due to the rapidly changing nature of science, research, known and unknown facts and internet. The Author and the publisher do not hold any responsibility for errors, omissions or contrary interpretation of the subject matter herein. This book is presented solely for motivational and informational purposes only.

Table of Contents

Introduction

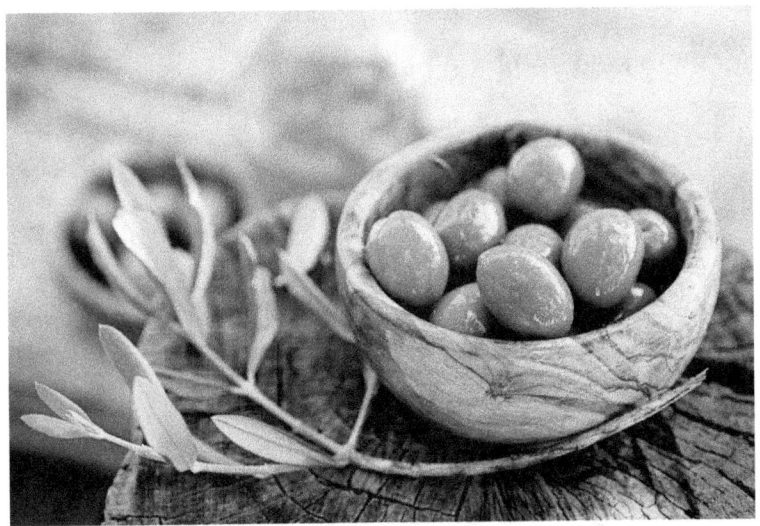

Have you been struggling to lose weight? Particularly stubborn body fat? If you feel like you have tried every diet in the book but nothing works, you probably haven't tried the belly fat diet. To lose stubborn belly fat you should focus on wholesome, nutritious foods and make sure to incorporate exercise into your weekly routine. Your diet should be rich in lean proteins, low-fat dairy products, high-fiber whole-grain carbohydrates and fresh vegetables. Some of the best foods to eat for burning belly fat include nuts, olive oil, fresh fruits, eggs, dried beans, whole grains, leafy green vegetables, fresh fish, avocado and green tea. In this book, you will receive a collection of 25 delicious recipes made with these foods to help you burn belly fat fast.

Organic Belly Fat Burner Recipes

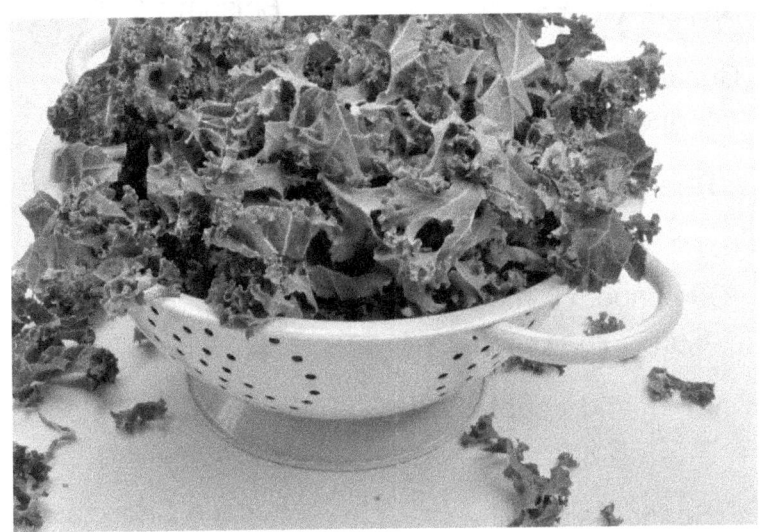

Recipes Included in this Book:

Egg White Veggie Omelet

Eggs Baked in Avocado

Sweet Potato Walnut Hash

Green Tea Avocado Smoothie

Mixed Veggie Frittata

Kale and Green Apple Smoothie

Fresh Fruit Salad with Mint

Homemade Strawberry Jam

Blueberry Banana Smoothie

Chilled Avocado Soup

Cucumber Red Onion and Dill Salad

Roasted Butternut Squash Soup

Cucumber, Tomato, Red Onion Salad

Chicken and Vegetable Soup

Spring Salad with Avocado and Mango

Cream of Broccoli Soup

Balsamic Spinach Salad with Avocado

Coconut-Crusted Tilapia

Balsamic Grilled Chicken Breast

Grilled Salmon with Mango Sauce

Rosemary Roasted Chicken

Poached Pears with Honey

Easy Coconut Flour Brownies

Avocado Chocolate Mousse

Flourless Almond Butter Cookies

Egg White Veggie Omelet

Eggs Baked in Avocado

Servings: 8

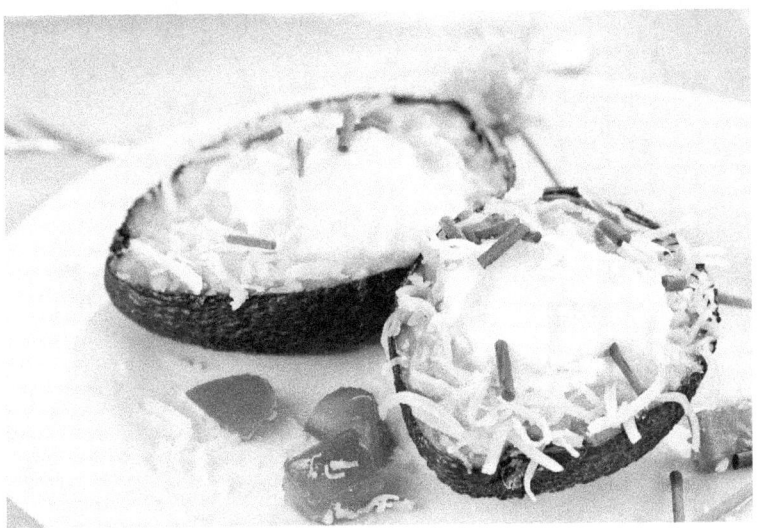

Ingredients:

4 ripe avocados

8 large eggs

Salt and pepper to taste

Fresh chopped chives

Instructions:

1. Preheat the oven to 425°F (220°C).
2. Cut the avocados in half lengthwise and remove the pits.
3. Scoop about 2 tablespoons of flesh from the middle of each avocado half and place them upright in a glass baking dish.
4. Crack an egg into each avocado half and sprinkle with salt and pepper.

5. Sprinkle with low-fat shredded cheese and bake 16 to 18 minutes until the egg is set.
6. Garnish with chopped chive to serve.

Sweet Potato Walnut Hash

Servings: 6

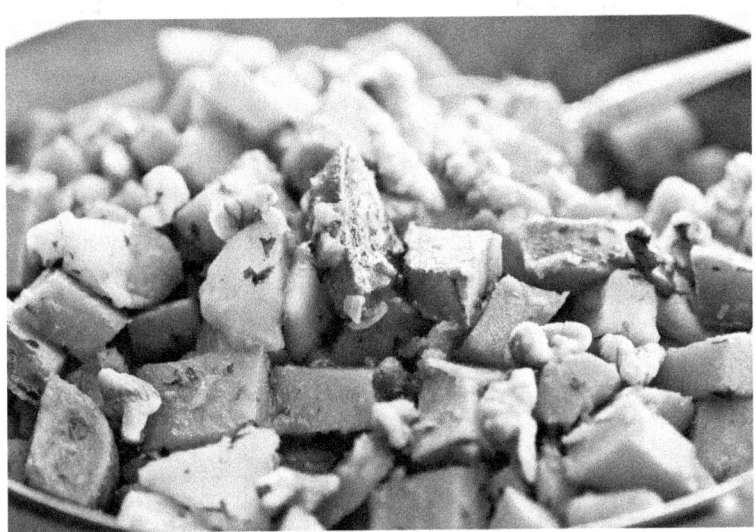

Ingredients:

2 tablespoons olive oil

1 large yellow onion, chopped

1 cup chopped carrots

1 cup chopped cauliflower florets

2 medium sweet potatoes, peeled and chopped

¼ cup fresh chopped parsley

¼ cup chopped walnuts

1 teaspoon chili powder

Salt and pepper to taste

Instructions:

1. Heat the oil in a large skillet over medium-high heat.
2. Add the onions, carrots, cauliflower and sweet potato.
3. Sauté for 6 minutes, stirring often, until the onion is translucent.
4. Add 2 tablespoons water then cover and let the vegetables steam for about 2 minutes.
5. Remove the lid and stir in the parsley, walnuts, chili powder, salt and pepper.
6. Cook for another 3 to 5 minutes until tender and browned.

Green Tea Avocado Smoothie

Servings: 1 to 2

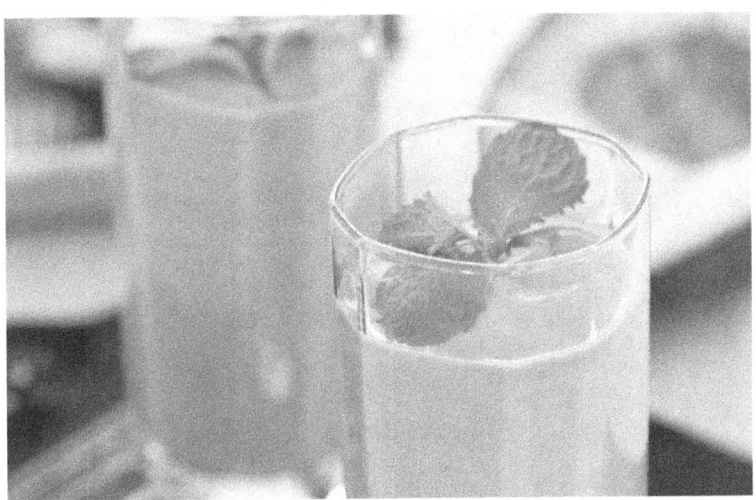

Ingredients:

1 medium ripe avocado, pitted and chopped

1 medium frozen banana, peeled and chopped

1 cup brewed green tea, chilled

½ cup non-fat Greek yogurt

1 teaspoon honey

Instructions:

1. Combine all of the ingredients in a high-speed blender.
2. Blend the mixture on high speed for 30 to 60 seconds until smooth.
3. Divide the smoothie among two glasses and serve immediately.

Mixed Veggie Frittata

Servings: 4 to 6

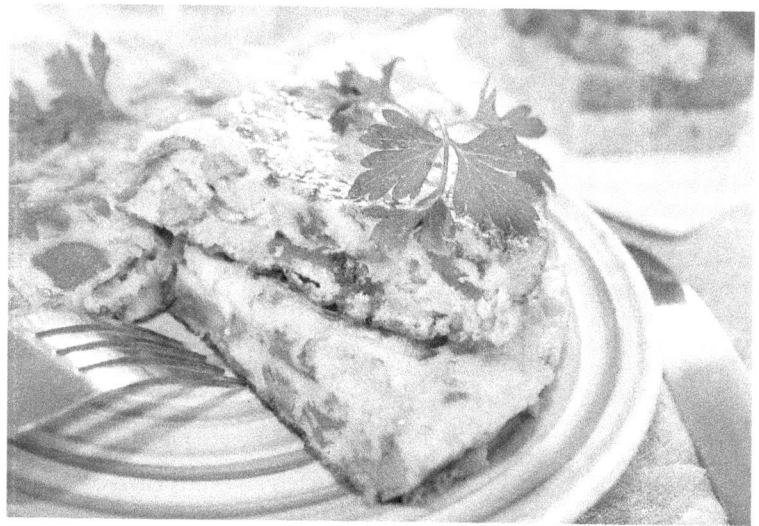

Ingredients:

1 tablespoon olive oil

1 small yellow onion, chopped

1 cup zucchini, peeled and diced

½ cup chopped broccoli florets

½ small red pepper, cored and diced

8 large eggs, whisked well

3 tablespoons water

1 tablespoon chopped chives

Salt and pepper to taste

½ cup reduced fat shredded cheddar cheese

Instructions:

1. Preheat the broiler in your oven to high heat.
2. Heat the oil in a large oven-proof skillet over medium heat.
3. Add the onion, zucchini, broccoli and red pepper – cook for 5 to 6 minutes until the vegetables are tender.
4. Whisk together the eggs, water, chives, salt and pepper.
5. Pour the egg mixture into the skillet and sprinkle with cheese.
6. Cook for 4 to 6 minutes until the eggs begin to set.
7. Transfer the skillet to the oven and broil for 2 minutes or so until the eggs are set and the cheese is melted.

Kale and Green Apple Smoothie

Servings: 1 to 2

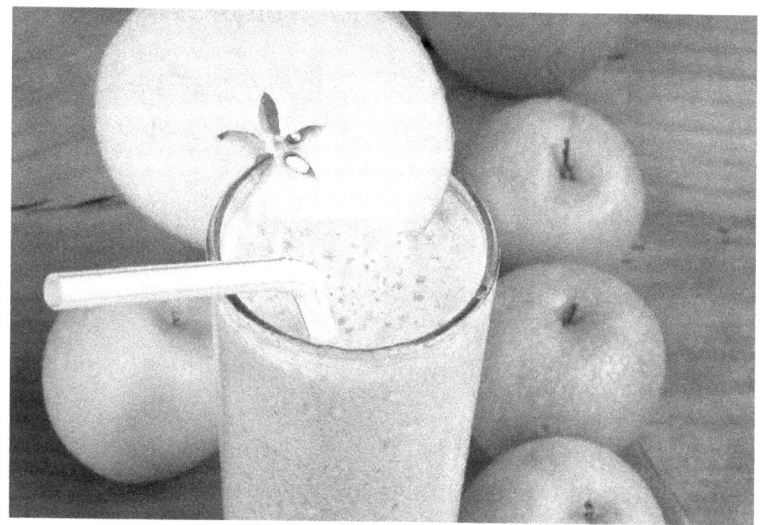

Ingredients:

1 large frozen banana, peeled and chopped

1 medium ripe apple, cored and chopped

1 cup skim milk

½ cup non-fat Greek yogurt

1 teaspoon honey

Pinch ground cinnamon

Instructions:

1. Combine all of the ingredients in a high-speed blender.
2. Blend the mixture on high speed for 30 to 60 seconds until smooth.

3. Divide the smoothie among two glasses and serve immediately.

Fresh Fruit Salad with Mint

Servings: 6 to 8

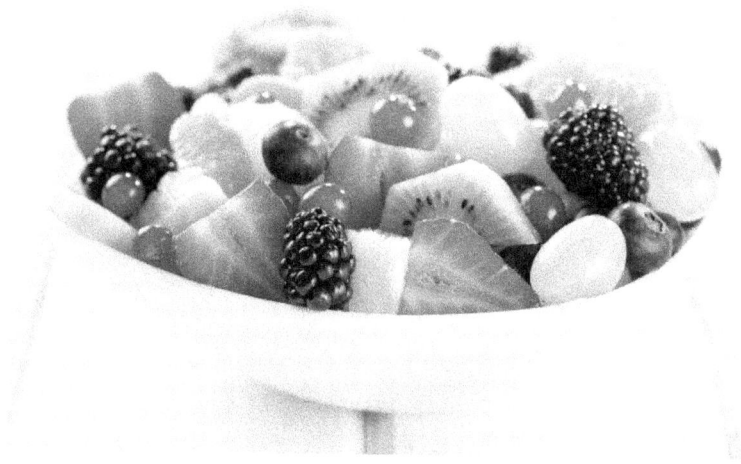

Ingredients:

1 ½ cups fresh sliced strawberries

1 cup fresh sliced pineapple

1 cup fresh blackberries

1 cup seedless green grapes

½ cup fresh blueberries

1 ripe kiwi, peeled and sliced

1 mandarin orange, peeled and chopped

Instructions:

1. Combine the fruit in a decorative serving bowl.
2. Toss in the mint and lime juice.
3. Chill until ready to serve.

Homemade Strawberry Jam

Servings: yields about 1 ½ cups

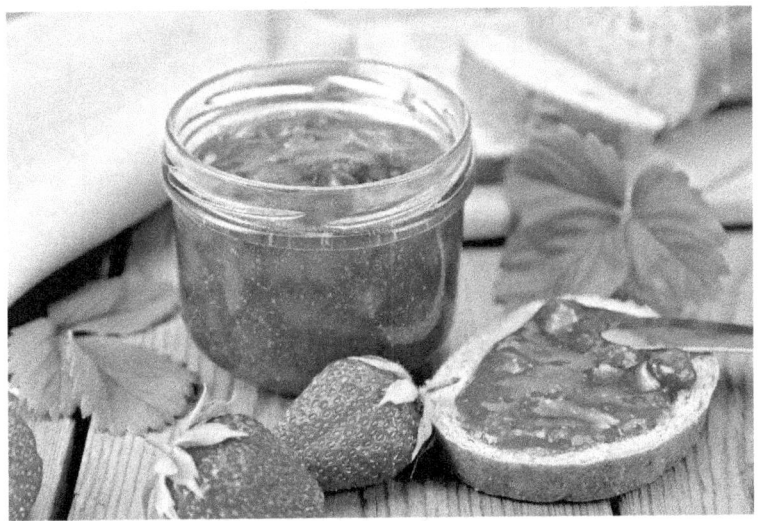

Ingredients:

1 lbs. fresh strawberries, sliced

2 tablespoons honey

1 tablespoon fresh lemon juice

Instructions:

1. Combine the strawberries, lemon juice and honey in a saucepan.
2. Bring to boil then simmer on medium-low for about 5 minutes.
3. Remove from heat and mash the berry mixture with a potato masher.
4. Return to heat and simmer on low for 20 minutes until thick.

5. Allow the jam to cool to room temperature then spoon into jars and chill overnight before using.

Blueberry Banana Smoothie

Servings: 1 to 2

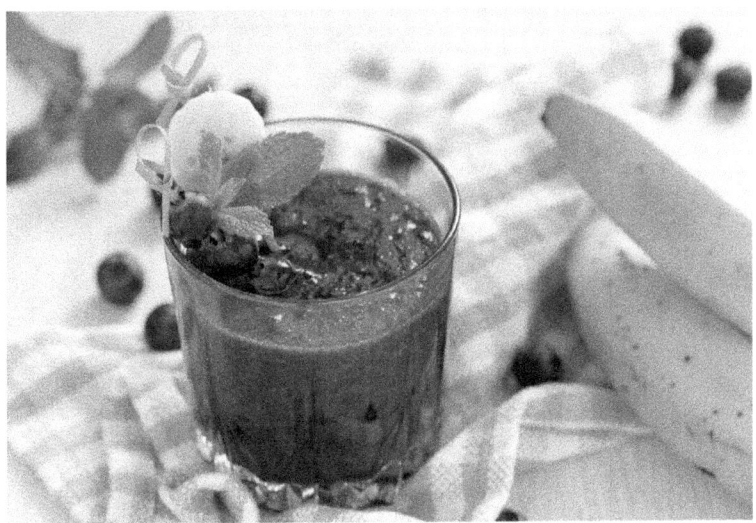

Ingredients:

1 ½ cups frozen blueberries

1 large frozen banana, peeled and chopped

1 cup non-fat Greek yogurt

½ cup skim milk

¼ cup ice cubes

Pinch ground cinnamon

Instructions:

1. Combine all of the ingredients in a high-speed blender.
2. Blend the mixture on high speed for 30 to 60 seconds until smooth.

3. Divide the smoothie among two glasses and serve immediately.

Chilled Avocado Soup

Servings: 6 to 8

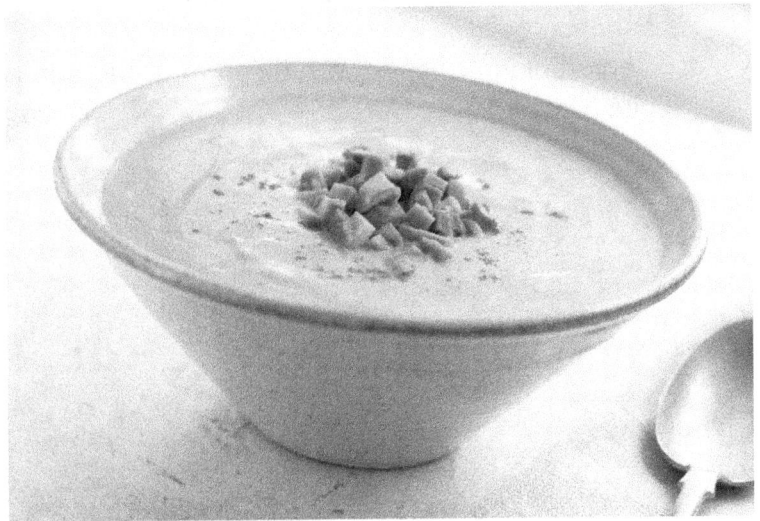

Ingredients:

4 large ripe avocado, pitted and chopped

1 small white onion, diced

3 cloves minced garlic

4 cups chicken broth or vegetable broth

2 cups cold water

½ cup fat-free sour cream

2 tablespoons fresh lemon juice

Salt and pepper to taste

Instructions:

1. Combine all of the ingredients in a food processor.

2. Blend the mixture until smooth and well combined then pour into a bowl.
3. Cover and chill for at least 6 hours before serving.
4. Serve cold garnished with diced avocado and a pinch of paprika.

Cucumber Red Onion and Dill Salad

Servings: 6

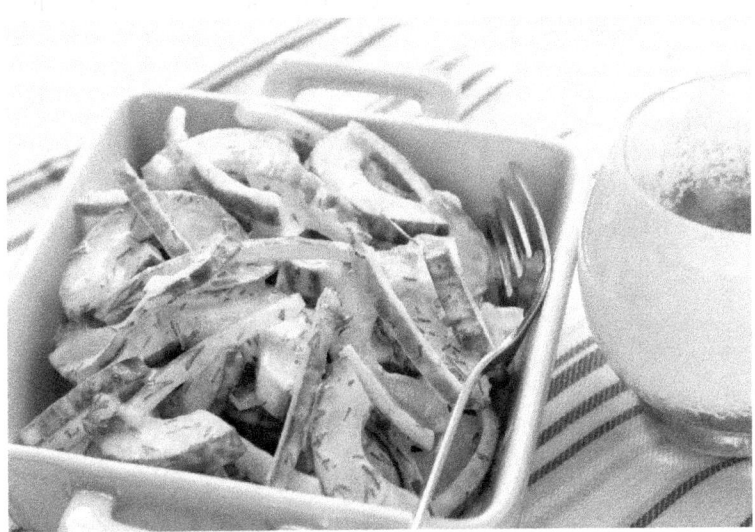

Ingredients:

1 large seedless cucumber, sliced thin

½ small red onion, sliced thin

3 tablespoons rice wine vinegar

1 tablespoon Dijon mustard

1 tablespoon fresh chopped dill

1 teaspoon honey

Salt and pepper to taste

Instructions:

1. Combine the cucumber and red onion in a salad bowl.

2. Whisk together the remaining ingredients in a separate bowl.
3. Toss the salad with the dressing then chill until ready to serve.

Roasted Butternut Squash Soup

Servings: 6

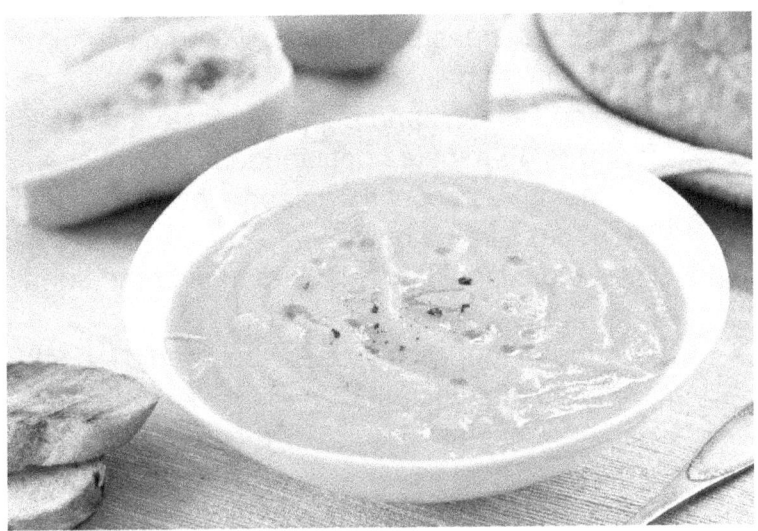

Ingredients:

2 medium butternut squash

Salt and pepper to taste

2 tablespoons olive oil

1 medium yellow onion, chopped

1 carrot, chopped

1 stalk celery, chopped

1 clove minced garlic

4 cups chicken broth or vegetable broth

½ teaspoon dried thyme

Instructions:

1. Preheat the oven to 350°F (180°C).
2. Cut the squashes in half and scoop out the seeds.
3. Brush the squash with olive oil then place them on a rimmed baking sheet.
4. Season with salt and pepper to taste then roast for 30 to 45 minutes until tender.
5. Let the squash cool then spoon the flesh out of the squash into a bowl.
6. Heat the oil in a large saucepan over medium heat.
7. Add the onion, carrot, celery and garlic – cook for 5 to 6 minutes.
8. Stir in the squash, broth, thyme, salt and pepper.
9. Bring to a boil then reduce heat and simmer for 15 minutes.
10. Puree the soup using an immersion blender then serve hot.

Cucumber, Tomato, Red Onion Salad

Servings: 6

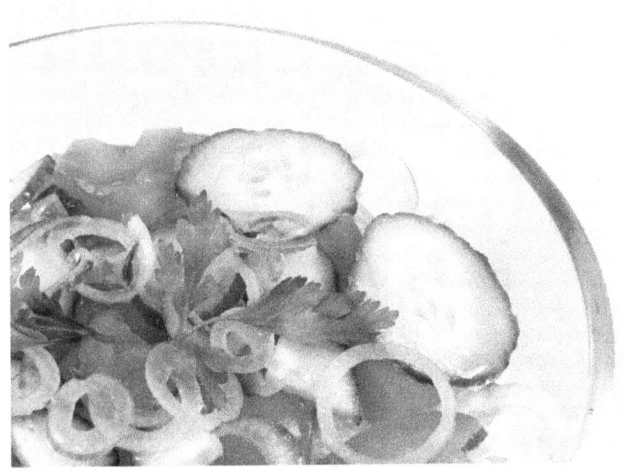

Ingredients:

2 large seedless cucumbers, sliced thin

3 large tomatoes, cored and chopped

1 small red onion, sliced thin

½ cup fresh chopped cilantro

¼ cup red wine vinegar

2 tablespoons olive oil

1 tablespoon honey

Salt and pepper to taste

Instructions:

1. Combine the cucumber, red onion and cilantro in a salad bowl.
2. Whisk together the remaining ingredients in a separate bowl.
3. Toss the salad with the dressing then chill until ready to serve.

Chicken and Vegetable Soup

Servings: 6 to 8

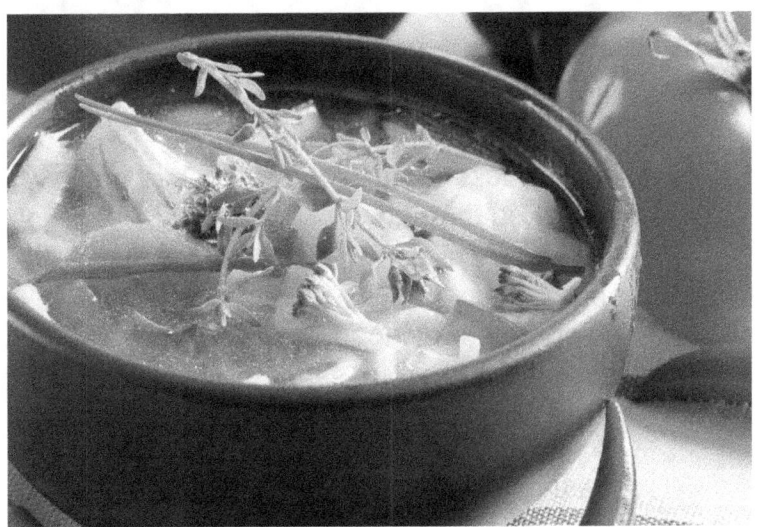

Ingredients:

4 cups water

2 cups chicken broth

1 lbs. boneless, skinless chicken, chopped

1 ½ tablespoons olive oil

1 medium yellow onion, diced

4 large carrots, peeled and sliced

2 medium stalks celery, sliced

1 tablespoon minced garlic

½ cup chopped broccoli florets

½ cup chopped cauliflower florets

Salt and pepper to taste

¼ cup fresh chopped parsley

Instructions:

1. Whisk together the broth and water in a large saucepan and bring to a simmer.
2. Add the chicken and cook for 5 to 6 minutes until cooked through.
3. Remove the chicken to a bowl using a slotted spoon.
4. In a separate saucepan, heat the oil over medium heat.
5. Add the onion, carrot, celery and garlic – cook for 5 to 6 minutes until tender.
6. Stir in the chicken cooking liquid along with the broccoli and cauliflower.
7. Season with salt and pepper to taste then simmer for 10 minutes.
8. Stir in the cooked chicken and fresh parsley then serve hot.

Spring Salad with Avocado and Mango

Servings: 4 to 6

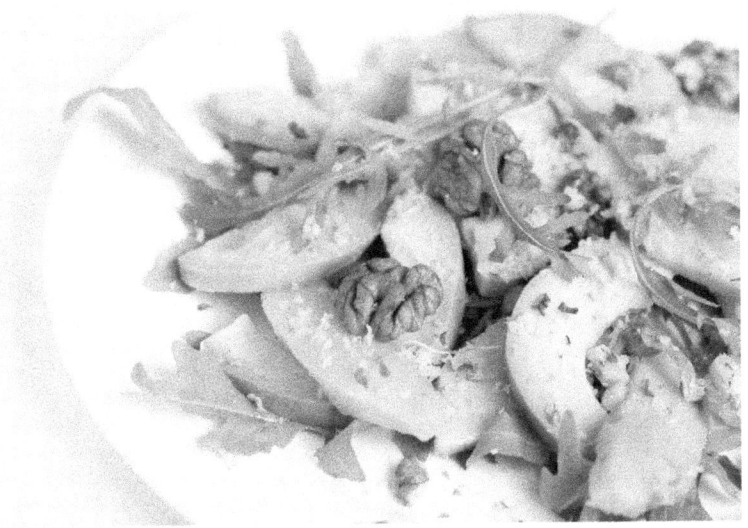

Ingredients:

6 cups fresh spring greens, packed

1 ½ cups fresh baby spinach

½ cup thinly sliced red onion

1 medium ripe avocado, pitted and sliced thin

1 medium ripe mango, pitted and sliced thin

½ cup chopped walnuts

Instructions:

1. Combine the spring greens, spinach and red onion in a salad bowl.
2. Top the salad with slices of avocado and mango.

3. Whisk together the remaining ingredients (except the walnuts) in a separate bowl.
4. Toss the salad with the dressing then chill until ready to serve – garnish with chopped walnuts.

Cream of Broccoli Soup

Servings: 6

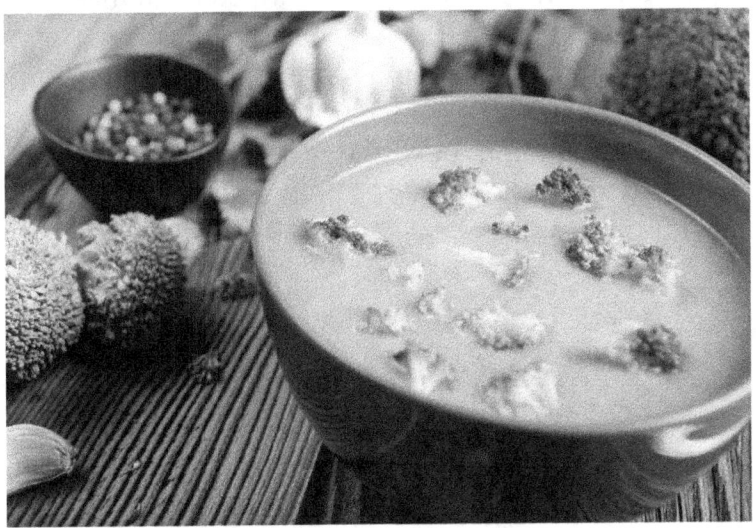

Ingredients:

1 tablespoon olive oil

1 medium yellow onion, chopped

8 cups fresh chopped broccoli florets

1 teaspoon minced garlic

4 cups vegetable broth (or chicken broth)

1 cup canned coconut milk

Salt and pepper to taste

Instructions:

1. Heat the olive oil in a large saucepan over medium-high heat and add the onion, broccoli, and garlic.

2. Cook for 6 to 8 minutes until the broccoli is tender-crisp.
3. Whisk in the vegetable broth, coconut milk, salt and pepper.
4. Bring to a boil then reduce heat and simmer for 20 minutes.
5. Remove from heat and puree the soup using an immersion blender. Serve hot.

Balsamic Spinach Salad with Avocado

Servings: 4

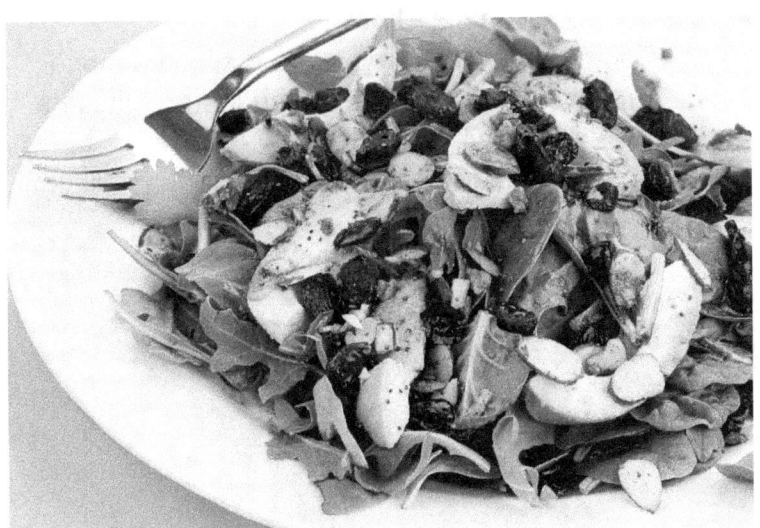

Ingredients:

6 cups fresh baby spinach, packed

1 cup sliced mushrooms

1 ripe avocado, pitted and sliced thin

½ cup seedless raisins

¼ cup sliced almonds

¼ cup extra-virgin olive oil

2 ½ tablespoons balsamic vinegar

1 tablespoon minced white onion

1 teaspoon honey

Pinch dry mustard powder

Instructions:

1. Combine the spinach, mushrooms, and avocado in a salad bowl.
2. Top the salad with raisins and sliced almonds.
3. Whisk together the remaining ingredients in a separate bowl.
4. Toss the salad with the dressing then chill until ready to serve.

Coconut-Crusted Tilapia

Servings: 4

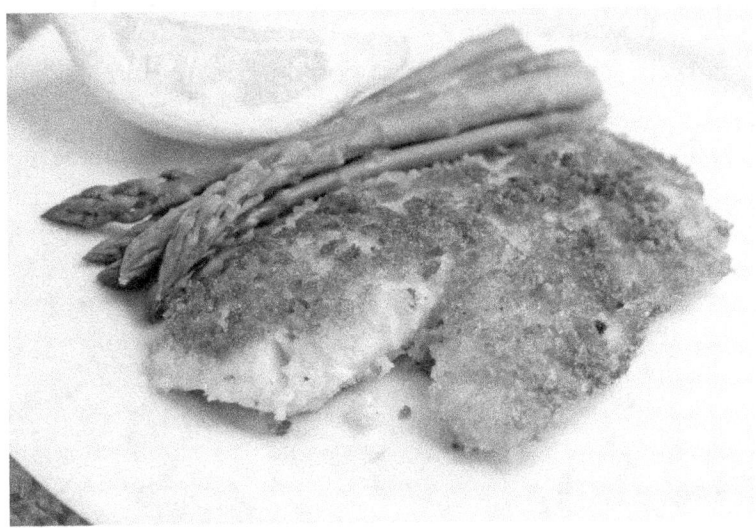

Ingredients:

4 (6-ounce) boneless tilapia fillets

1 to 2 tablespoons olive oil

Pinch chili powder

Salt and pepper to taste

¼ cup almond flour

¼ cup unsweetened shredded coconut

Lemon wedges

Instructions:

1. Preheat the oven to 350°F (180°C) and line a baking sheet with foil.

2. Brush the fillets with olive oil and season with chili powder, salt and pepper to taste.
3. Combine the almond flour and coconut in a bowl.
4. Place the fillets on the baking sheet and top with the coconut mixture.
5. Bake for 12 to 15 minutes until the flesh flakes easily with a fork.
6. Serve hot with lemon wedges.

Balsamic Grilled Chicken Breast

Servings: 6 to 8

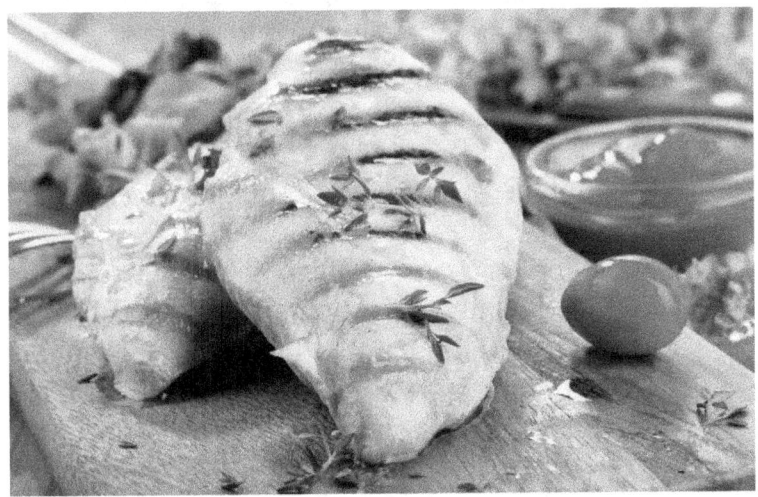

Ingredients:

8 boneless, skinless chicken breast halves

¾ cup balsamic vinegar

1/3 cup chicken broth

½ cup diced scallions

1 tablespoon minced garlic

1 teaspoon dry mustard powder

Salt and pepper to taste

Olive oil, as needed

Instructions:

1. Place the chicken in a large zippered freezer bag.

2. Whisk together the chicken broth, balsamic vinegar, scallions, garlic, and mustard – season with salt and pepper to taste.
3. Pour the marinade into the bag and toss with the chicken to coat.
4. Chill the chicken in the marinade for about 24 hours.
5. Preheat the grill to medium-high heat and brush the grates with olive oil.
6. Place the chicken breasts on the grill and cook for 5 to 6 minutes on each side, basting with the marinade, until cooked through.
7. Transfer the chicken to a cutting board and let rest for 5 minutes before slicing to serve.

Grilled Salmon with Mango Sauce

Servings: 6

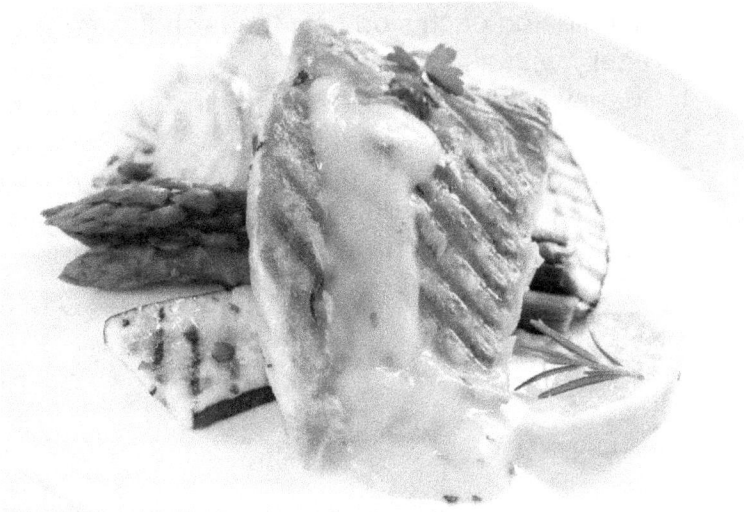

Ingredients:

6 (6-ounce) boneless salmon fillets

2 tablespoons olive oil

Salt and pepper to taste

1 large ripe mango, pitted and chopped

½ cup canned coconut milk

¼ cup fresh chopped cilantro

2 tablespoons fresh lime juice

Pinch salt

Instructions:

1. Preheat the grill to medium-high heat and brush the grates with olive oil.

2. Brush the salmon fillets with olive oil and season with salt and pepper to taste.
3. Place the fillets on the grill and cook for 4 to 5 minutes on each side until the flesh flakes easily with a fork.
4. Meanwhile, combine the remaining ingredients in a food processor or blender.
5. Blend on high speed until smooth and well combined then drizzle over the grilled salmon to serve.

Rosemary Roasted Chicken

Servings: 6 to 8

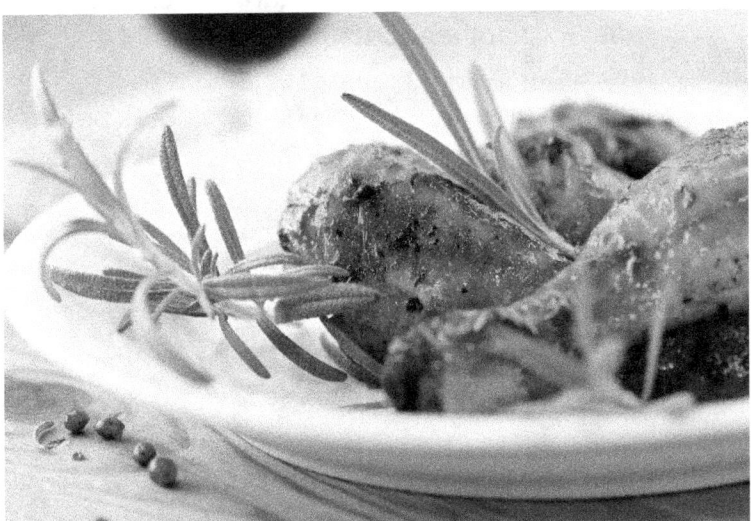

Ingredients:

2 tablespoons olive oil

2 ½ lbs. bone-in chicken thighs and drumsticks

Salt and pepper to taste

2 medium onions, sliced

Instructions:

1. Preheat the oven to 400°F (205°C).
2. Heat the oil in a large skillet over medium-high heat.
3. Add the chicken and season with salt and pepper to taste – cook for 2 to 3 minutes on each side until browned.
4. Transfer the chicken to a glass baking dish and top with the onions.

5. Season with salt and pepper to taste and sprinkle with rosemary.
6. Roast for 30 minutes then turn the chicken and roast for another 25 to 30 minutes until the juices run clear.
7. Let the chicken rest for 5 to 10 minutes before serving.

Poached Pears with Honey

Servings: 4 to 6

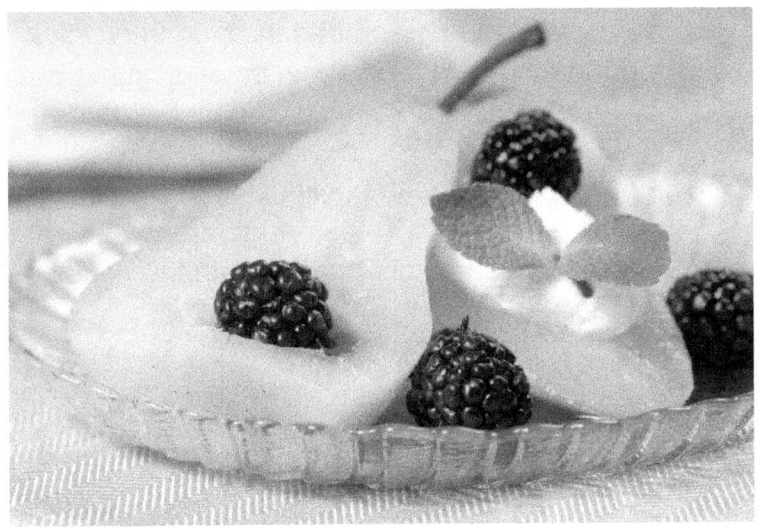

Ingredients:

5 ripe pears

4 ½ cups water

½ cup raw honey

1 teaspoon whole cloves

3 inches fresh ginger, peeled and sliced

1 (4-inch) cinnamon stick, broken in half

Instructions:

1. Peel the pears and cut them in half, top to bottom, leaving the stems in place.
2. Use a melon baller or spoon to cut out the core from each half.

3. Combine the water and honey in a saucepan and bring to boil over high heat.
4. Whisk until the honey is dissolved then stir in the cloves, ginger and add the cinnamon stick.
5. Add the pears to the saucepan and simmer, covered, for 22 to 25 minutes until the pears are fork-tender.
6. Pour the pears (with the liquid) into a plastic container and chill in the refrigerator overnight.
7. Serve the pears cold drizzled with the honey liquid.

Easy Coconut Flour Brownies

Servings: 14 to 16

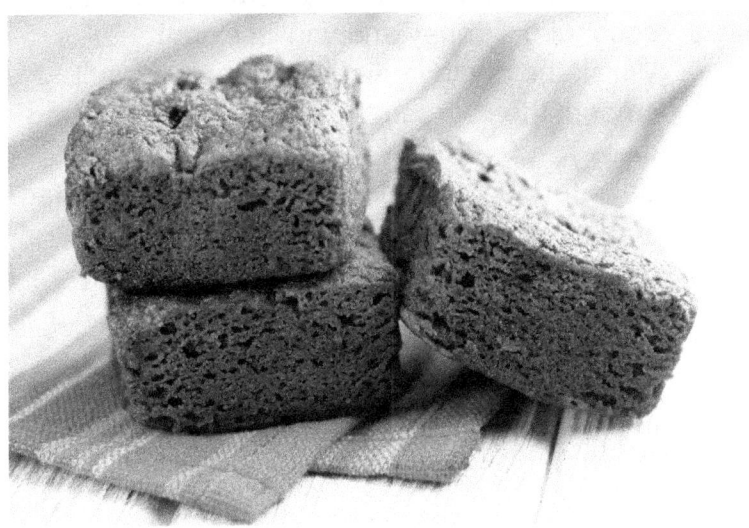

Ingredients:

½ cup coconut flour, sifted

½ cup plus 1 tablespoon unsweetened cocoa powder

¾ teaspoon baking soda

Pinch salt

3 large eggs, whisked well

2/3 cups coconut oil, melted

½ cup raw honey

2 teaspoons vanilla extract

Instructions:

1. Preheat the oven to 300°F (150°C) and grease a square glass baking dish.

2. Whisk together the coconut flour, cocoa powder, baking soda and salt.
3. In a separate bowl, beat together the eggs, coconut oil, honey and vanilla extract.
4. Whisk the dry ingredients into the wet until smooth then spread the batter in the prepared dish.
5. Bake for 30 to 35 minutes until a knife inserted in the center comes out clean.
6. Let the brownies cool completely before cutting.

Avocado Chocolate Mousse

Servings: 6 to 8

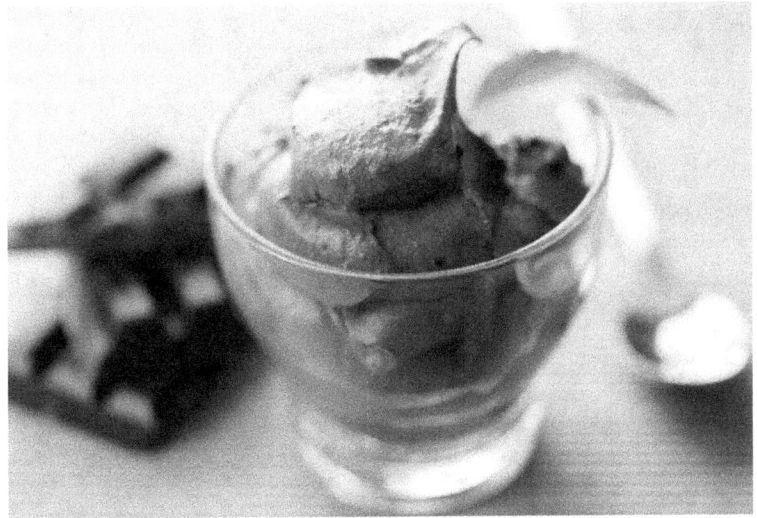

Ingredients:

4 small ripe avocado, pitted and chopped

½ cup plus 2 tablespoons canned coconut milk

1/3 cup raw honey

1/3 cup unsweetened cocoa powder

1 ¼ teaspoon vanilla extract

Pinch salt

Instructions:

1. Combine the ingredients in a food processor.
2. Blend on high speed until the mixture is smooth and well combined.
3. Spoon into dessert cups then chill for at least 1 hour before serving.

Flourless Almond Butter Cookies

Servings: yields about 2 dozen

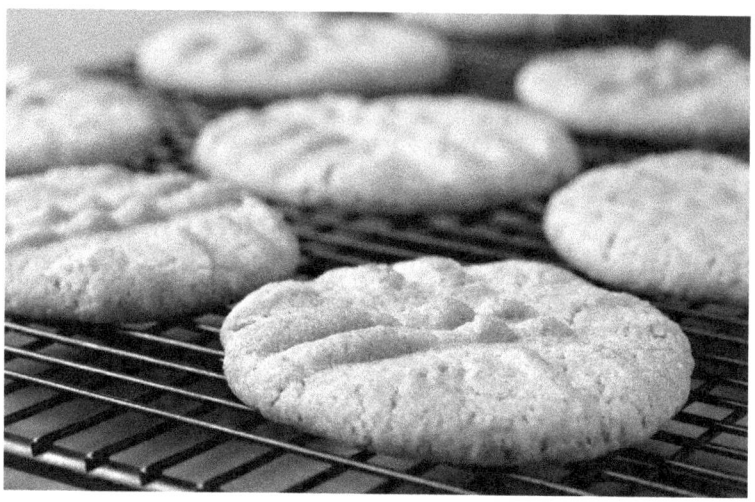

Ingredients:

1 cup smooth almond butter

1 cup coconut sugar

1 large egg, whisked

1 ¼ teaspoon baking soda

1 teaspoon vanilla extract

Instructions:

1. Preheat the oven to 350°F (180°C) and line two baking sheets with parchment.
2. Combine the almond butter, sugar, egg, baking soda and vanilla in a mixing bowl.
3. Whisk until well combined in a sticky dough.
4. Pinch off pieces of the dough and roll it into 1-inch balls by hand.

5. Place the dough balls on the baking sheet, spacing them 1 inch apart.
6. Flatten the cookies with a fork then bake for 10 to 12 minutes until the edges are just browned.
7. Cool the cookies for 5 minutes on the baking sheet then transfer to a wire rack to cool completely.

Conclusion

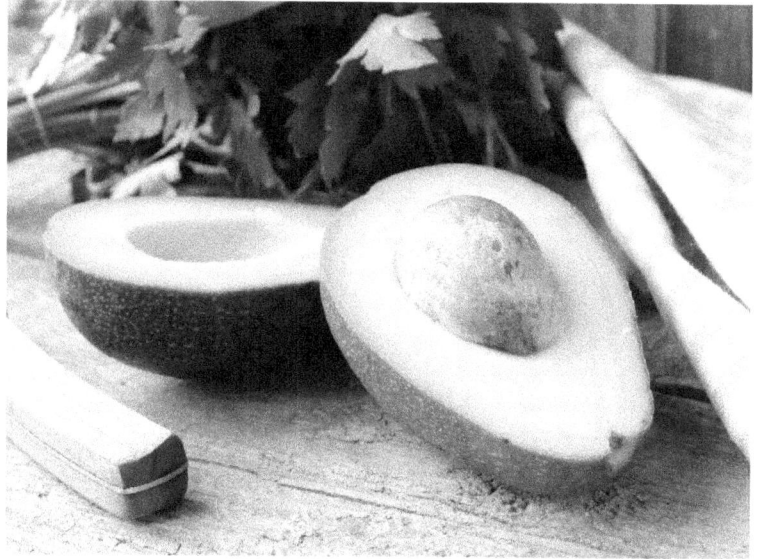

If you are tired to carrying around stubborn belly fat, this is the perfect diet for you. This diet is rich in lean proteins, low-fat dairy products, fresh vegetables, and whole-grain carbohydrates. To get started burning belly fat fast, pick a recipe from this book and get cooking. You will love every recipe in this book and you might be surprised just how quickly you start to burn stubborn belly fat.

www.ingramcontent.com/pod-product-compliance
Lightning Source LLC
Chambersburg PA
CBHW070336290526
45791CB00003B/1350